THE VEGAN WARRIOR

BENEFITS OF A VEGAN DIET FOR ACTIVE SPORTS

PEOPLE AND ASPIRING ATHLETES

By

BASTIEN DARROW

Table of Contents

Introduction

I want to thank you and congratulate you for downloading the book, "The Vegan Warrior: Benefits Of A Vegan Diet For Active Sports People And Aspiring Athletes".

This book contains proven steps and strategies on how to harness the power of a vegan diet. It will discuss what a vegan diet is, how to become vegan, the most popular reasons to become a vegan, famous athletes who are proudly vegan, and also talk about some of the supplements that are available for vegans.

Vegans come from all walks of life. They are of every nationality and every race. Being a vegan is more of a philosophy and lifestyle choice than it is an actual diet. The reasons for becoming a vegan could be to obtain better health, for environmental reasons, or due to the ethical concerns surrounding animal rights. Whatever the reasons may be for you, there is overwhelming evidence that shows how much healthier a vegan diet is for everyone, not just aspiring athletes. Some of the world's best athletes are vegan. This would not have been possible if a vegan diet had not met the needs of their bodies and increased their performance.

While many believe that a completely vegan diet is a new concept, it literally goes back almost until the dawn of human time. Everyone is familiar with the Roman Gladiators. These athletes fought wild boars, lions, and each other in arenas cheered on by thousands of people. Discoveries in recent years have shown that the diet for the majority of Gladiators was vegan. Even back then they were able to see the benefits that a vegan diet had on their performance while training and while fighting inside the arena.

According to statistics, the number of vegans in the US is increasing year by year. Numbers in 2006 reported that 1.4% of all people living in the U.S. were vegan. In 2008, that number dropped slightly to 0.5%. Another increase was reported in 2009, with final numbers showing 1%. By 2012 that number had doubled, or 2%. Skipping ahead to 2014 there has been a significant increase of vegans in the US. A Harris Interactive study reported that 5% of people living in the US were fully vegan or in the process of making the switch. These numbers are only expected to increase as more people discover all of the benefits that being vegan offers.

Chapter 1- What Is a Vegan Diet

Veganism is one type of a vegetarian diet. Exclusions for those who are vegan include any meat, dairy products, eggs, and any other ingredients that are derived from animals. A growing number of people who follow a vegan diet also do not eat any type of food that has been processed using any kind of animal products, including certain types of wines and white sugar that has been refined. The actual term "vegan" can either refer to the diet itself or a person who has adopted this style of eating.

What Do Vegans Eat?

To those who are not familiar with Veganism, this is the most common question that is asked. Many people have visions of a plate of salad night after night for the rest of their lives. In reality, a vegan diet is quite diverse. It includes fruits, vegetables, legumes, beans, and all grains. Think of the infinite combination of delicious meals that can be made from these ingredients! There are also vegan options for most of the popular dishes people enjoy eating. Some common examples include vegan mayonnaise, vegan cheese, vegan ice cream, vegan hot dogs, vegan pizza, and tons of others.

If you were to ask a vegan if they feel restricted by choosing to follow their diet, their answer would always be a resounding, "No".

How to Become a Vegan

Once you have made the decision to become a vegan, it can be difficult to know where to start. Do you shun all animal related products right away? Do you ease into it gently? The simple answer is that it will completely depend on you. While some people may find the switch a simple matter, others may struggle with their decision.

For people who find the commitment difficult in the beginning, one painless way to start is by becoming a vegetarian first. Once you have the basics of vegetarianism down pat, slowly omit dairy and eggs. There is no wrong or right way to go about becoming a vegan so do what feels right for you. In order to keep yourself on the right track, keep the reasons that you chose to become vegan in mind in the first place and the goals that you have set for yourself.

Chapter 2- Main Reasons for Making the Switch to Veganism

Vegans are strictly against testing done on animals. They avoid all companies who test their products on animals before they are approved for human use. This includes cleaning products, skin care products, and a host of others. There are three main reasons why most people choose to become vegan. Some vegans are interested in only one reason while others make the switch for all three.

- **Animal Rights**: Even though the use of eggs or dairy products would not result in the death of an animal, vegans still avoid them at all costs. The main reason for this is the belief that animals have the right to live their lives without interference from humans. Secondary to this reason is the knowledge that dairy cows and laying chickens are commonly slaughtered once their productivity begins to decrease as they get older. A mass slaughter of animals would still occur even if humans only ate eggs and dairy products because cockerels and bulls are considered to be unproductive animals. All vegans believe that their diet is the only way to live a truly cruelty-free existence.

- **Health:** Studies have shown that eating animal protein and animal fats increase the average person's risk of heart disease, hypertension, rheumatoid arthritis, diabetes, cancer, and a vast number of other conditions and illnesses. Cow's milk contains protein and fat content that is extremely different from the milk of humans. Humans were not designed to consume the milk of another species. The mainstays of a vegan diet - legumes, fruits, vegetables, and whole grains are low in fat, and contain no cholesterol. Each of them is also high in a variety of nutrients and soluble fiber.

- **Environment:** The effects of livestock farming are devastating on planet Earth. It is extremely inefficient since the production of meat and animal products uses up an immense amount of water, grains, fertilizers, land, and various other resources.

These resources could be used more effectively to feed humans. Topsoil erosion is occurring at an accelerated rate because of the farmer's pursuit of higher and higher yields. Another thing to consider is the amount of pollution found in rivers and the groundwater due to animal waste.

Chapter 3- The Top 10 Famous Vegan Athletes

Athletes are respected throughout the world for their skills, stamina, and abilities. Their bodies require a huge amount of fuel, vitamins, and minerals in order to perform effectively both on and off their field of choice. If Veganism was not healthy, how could these athletes make it through their training and competitions? The answer is that they could not.

The typical diet of an athlete is changing. History is beginning to show that those who have a competitive spirit are no longer meat-eaters, but "conscious eaters." Many historic Olympians have made the choice to keep a vegetarian or vegan lifestyle, or they have decided to change from a diet that utilized meats for protein into one that is protein-rich from plant-based sources. There are thousands of celebrities and athletes who have made the switch to a vegan diet. Here are the top 10 famous vegan athletes who are able to outperform the competition:

1. Brendan Brazier: Brendan is one of the top athletes in the world. A Canadian professional Ironman triathlete. He has gained notoriety by winning the Canadian 50 km Ultra Marathon Championships twice. He has placed both 2nd and 3rd at the Royal Victoria two years in a row. Added to that is a

3rd place medal at the National Long-Course Triathlon Championships.

Brendan made the switch to becoming a vegan after he had tried several different types of diets and found that he performed best on a vegan diet. Along with being a successful consultant in performance nutrition, he is the bestselling author of the book series *Thrive,* and the formulator of Vega, an award-winning line of plant-based nutritional products. VegNews Magazine listed Brendan as one of the "Top 25 Most Fascinating Vegetarians" and named him "Favorite Athlete" for two years running.

"I formulated Vega using the highest quality, least processed, plant-based Superfoods available. Armed with Vega, you will no longer need to compromise between whole food goodness and fast food convenience. To me, Vega is a way of life. I hope you enjoy it as much as I do." ~ Brendan Brazier

"When we bite into food, part of the environment becomes part of us," ~ Brendan Brazier

2. Robert Cheeke: Anyone who believes they need to eat animal protein to be a world-class bodybuilder has never met Robert. Not only is he the founder and president of Vegan Body Builder, but he has been a vegan competitor since 1995. He began his athletic career at Oregon State University with cross-country running, but it wasn't long before he developed an interest in strength training and weight-lifting. He took home the gold medal at the INBA Northwester USA Overall Novice Bodybuilding Championship in 2005, and he has also been ranked as one of the most influential vegan athletes in the world by VegNews. A documentary titled, "*Vegan Fitness: Built Naturally*" was released in 2006 by Robert and also featured top vegan athletes Tonya Kay and Brendan Brazier. When he is not busy training and competing, Robert travels throughout the United States promoting his books and doing motivational speaking.

"I grew up on a farm and developed an appreciation for farm animals similar to the respect and appreciation someone might have for a dog or a cat. Given this perspective of farm animals and my closeness to them through my involvement in 4-H, raising them as pets, it seemed fitting to stop eating my animal friends. I no longer wanted to contribute to animal cruelty and suffering and decided to go vegan." ~ Robert Cheeke

"A vegan diet/lifestyle is very conducive to success in athletics because plant-based whole foods provide the best sources of nutrition, coming from their original forms. The nutritional components we need to thrive are vitamins, minerals, amino acids, fatty acids and glucose and those all come in their

original and best forms from fruits, vegetables, nuts, grains, seeds and legumes." ~ Robert Cheeke

3. Robert Hazeley: Robert's career began with professional bodybuilding in 1971. Turning 60 in 2015, he was forced to give up his sport in the 1990s after several operations on his tendon injuries that required the use of painkillers on a regular basis. After an introduction to a vegan diet by his friend and gym owner, Dave Howe, he has never looked back. The recovery that he experienced by changing to a vegan diet is nearly miraculous. Painkillers are now a thing of the past and he takes a 30 mile "stroll" once per week.

He began training for contests again in 1994, but this time as a vegan. On stage in 1995, Robert weighed 184lbs/83Kg - that is 6 pounds heavier than he'd manage to achieve eating meat! During 2005, Robert placed 3rd in Mr. England, 4th in the British Championship, 2nd in Mr. Wales, 2nd in Mr. Britain, and 6th in World Power Lifting. Robert changes his diet to coincide with his increased needs when preparing for competitions or "bulking up".

"I went vegan in the 1990s and that was on health grounds. I started bodybuilding back in 1971 and was experiencing a number of health problems, especially with my knees. Going vegan made a lot of sense on paper and in practice was

instrumental in improving my all performance. It was the turning point for me in so many ways." ~ Robert Hazeley

"Remaining on a vegan diet has improved my training ability and intensity, kept my stamina high, and has helped to keep me free from injuries" ~ Robert Hazeley

4. Georges Laraque: Professional NHL player Georges won the "Best Fighter" award in 2003 from The Hockey News. He was named "The Number One Enforcer" by Sports Illustrated in 2008. He is best known for being a defenseman, but his offense is also worth looking at. During a game against the LA Kings in 2000, Georges managed to score the elusive hat trick. Playing for teams such as the Pittsburgh Penguins, Phoenix Coyotes, and the Edmonton Oilers, he retired from the NHL in 2010 when the Montreal Canadiens bought out the remainder of his free-agent contract.

After leaving the world of professional hockey, he turned to politics. In February of 2010 he became a member of the Green Party of Canada and was named as one of their deputy leaders in July of that year. Georges became a vegan in 2009, protesting against the cruelty of the meat industry. He vocally supports many animal charities.

"I became vegan immediately after watching the documentary Earthling. I have never felt better physically and mentally, and wished I had done that 20 years ago." ~ Georges Laraque

"The fact that I have been vegan now for just over two years is breaking the stereotype that "Real men eat meat", and there're

many other athletes like me that are big, vegan and successful. I have not lost any muscle mass at all and actually got stronger, so the meat quote is just a dumb way for people not wanting that lifestyle." ~ Georges Laraque

5. Carl Lewis: Almost everyone is familiar with this Olympic athlete who is likely one of the most famous people in the world. In the 1984 Olympic Games, he took home an impressive 10 medals, 9 of which were gold. He chose to become a vegan in 1990. His resume is long and distinguished. He holds 10 World Championship medals and 8 of these are gold. He has received top rankings in both the 200 meter and the 100 meter sprinting events, along with several long jump events. Athlete of the Year was given to him in 1982, 1983, and 1984. He also holds the world record for relays. Additionally, he has been voted "Olympian of the Century" by Sports Illustrated and "Sportsman of the Century" by the International Olympic Committee. Carl is also the only man in the world to defend an Olympic long jump or 100 meter title successfully.

"I've found that a person does not need protein from meat to be a successful athlete. In fact, my best year of track competition was the first year I ate a vegan diet. Moreover, by continuing to eat a vegan diet, my weight is under control, I like the way I look. (I know that sounds vain, but all of us want

to like the way we look.) I enjoy eating more, and I feel great."
~ Carl Lewis

"It's a myth that muscles, strength, and endurance require the consumption of large quantities of animal-based foods. This myth began before anyone even talked about protein." He ended his introduction with, "Your body is your temple. If you nourish it properly, it will be good to you, and you will increase its longevity." ~ Carl Lewis

6. Jack Lindquist: Before becoming a competitive cyclist, Jack had formerly worked in the defense industry and was an Aerospace student. He found the idea of creating weapons distasteful, so he became a bike messenger and later started to compete in various events. Eventually, he won his first medal at New York City's Puma Velocity Race in 2007. This gave him notoriety worldwide, and he now sits on the U.S. National Developmental Team. His most recent first place win was in 2011 during the Mothballs Criterium. Jack became vegan in 2005 after many discussions with fellow competitors and friends. It was a logical path to follow because he was an avid environmentalist and compassionate person already.

"It was truly a 'eureka' moment. I had a bunch of friends that were vegan while I still ate meat and dairy. I have always been a bit of an environmentalist, walking or riding my bike instead

of driving, etc, and after talking with them for a bit, and realizing how horribly my current habits affected the planet and animals, which I've always loved, I went vegan overnight….A friend asked me what the difference was between my dog, The Reverend, and a cow. I didn't have an answer, and that was that. I had a lot of friends that are vegan, including a nutritionist and registered dietician, so that helped me a lot." ~ Jack Lindquist

"I feel that my vegan diet allows me to recover quicker than I would on a similar, meat based diet. I have more energy, and can get back on my feet quicker, and with less soreness after a particularly brutal workout. When other cyclists, find out that I don't eat meat they are usually a little shocked. I don't 'look vegan'; I'm not skinny and lethargic, and I'm muscular and well proportioned." ~ Jack Lindquist

7. **Mike Mahler:** Since 1997 this kettlebell instructor and strength coach has been vegan. Among the famous athletes he trained one of them was former UFC light heavyweight champion, Frank Shamrock. His unbelievable strength was measured as followed: 500 pounds of deadlifting, 6 reps of 315 pound bench press, one-arm kettlebell snatch, 17 reps at 105 pounds, one-arm kettlebell military press, 10 reps at 97 pounds, and double kettlebell clean and military press, 10 reps using two 88 pound bells.

He is in demand all over the world for the workshops that he teaches. Mike is also a best-selling author and has produced a couple of DVDs. He is a frequent contributing writer to Vegsource, Testosterone, Ironman, Hardcore Muscle, Industry, and Exercise Magazine for Men.

"I love animals and eating a vegan diet plays a big role in my spiritual and ethical values. I like knowing that I can be strong, healthy and have an optimal
hormone profile on a vegan diet. I do not have to compromise my values. I thrive very well on vegan food and feel that I am able to extract a great deal of energy from the food I eat without having to utilize a great deal of energy. I wake up refreshed and ready to go and attack workouts and projects."
~ Mike Mahler

"I think it is important to avoid overly processed food. Stick to real vegan food and get complete protein from combining legumes with nuts and seeds. This combination has a nice balance of protein, fat, and low Glycemic carbohydrates. Make sure to have a salad every day and eat some raw fruits and veggies. Coconut oil is a must for vegans as it is loaded with MCFA for energy and is a saturated fat that helps with hormone optimization and a healthy metabolism." ~ Mike Mahler

8. Patrick J. Neshek: After reading *The China Study*, the relief pitcher of the Minnesota Twins became vegan in 2007. He credits the book with giving him the opportunity to discover how powerful the vegan diet is and how it changed his career for the better. Both Baseball Tonight and SportsCenter have commented on the strength he has while pitching. During the 2007 year, he was awarded the Dick Siebert Award for Upper Midwest Player of the Year by Minnesota.

"I decided to become a vegan and get rid of all the animal products -- meat and dairy. At first, it was basically just for the health benefits -- I was intrigued by the 2005 season when I cut a lot of that stuff out and got a lot better. It really changed my career, and I thought, 'This might be something that helps me take my career to the next level.' And it wasn't the main reason, but I like knowing everything I eat was served in a humane way." ~ Patrick J. Neshek

"I'll have a granola and fruit smoothie in the morning, and for protein I'll throw a rice protein substitute in my smoothie...I just got my blood work back, and everything checked out perfect. I think you have that in the back of your mind that maybe you're missing something [because of eating vegan]. It's pretty neat to know you don't have to use animal products and can still function -- most of my results had improved" ~ Patrick J. Neshek

9. Fiona Oakes: Fiona became a vegan during her teen years, even though she had stopped eating meat at the age of 6. She is a retained firefighter and runs an animal sanctuary in Essex, UK that cares for more than 400 animals, including dogs, sheep, pigs, and horses.

She became the Essex County Marathon Champion in 2007, a record that is still standing today. She competes in marathons throughout the world at the international level and has placed in the top 10 in both Florence and Amsterdam. Some of her other career highlights include being the fastest woman on record to ever complete marathons on every single continent and the North Pole. She has also set the world record in the Guinness Books for the fastest times in those races. Additionally, she broke two of her own world records when she ran the Rio Marathon in 2014.

"I like to encourage people to think about Veganism in a positive way. I try to break down stereotypes and myths attached to Veganism by my actions. I am one of only 800 female fire-fighters in the UK - a job which people don't expect to see a female doing, let alone a vegan one. I run endurance events, a thing which people don't think you can do if you are a 'weak vegan'." ~ Fiona Oakes

"The thought of saving the lives of innocent animals is my main motivation to be so committed and sacrifice so much for my training. To lead by example and to show people that a vegan diet is in no way prohibitive to sporting excellence. If by doing this I can convince just one person (hopefully more) to consider a vegan lifestyle then this is all the reward I need for my efforts." ~ Fiona Oakes

10. Amanda Reister: Amanda is a certified USA boxing judge, officiant, and coach. By age 16, she had entered into the Chicago Golden Gloves, an annual competition for amateurs, and at 17 she started boxing at the national level. At 18, she was rated number two in the entire US. She retired after ten years of boxing with an incredible total of four Chicago Golden Gloves titles. Then she started bodybuilding and coaching. In 2011, she placed 1st in the Natural North America Bodybuilding Championships and first runner up in the Windy City Classic Natural Bodybuilding Championship.

She became a full vegan at age 29, making the switch from a vegetarian diet. Immediately after making the switch she was delighted to notice a large improvement in her overall health and energy level. She follows a highly structured diet, eating 25 grams of protein and raw green veggies every three hours. She is also fanatical about drinking a minimum of three gallons of water per day.

"I decided to become a vegan because it was the right thing to do. I don't believe God put these precious creatures here for us to exploit and murder. As a cancer survivor, I appreciate that a plant-based diet is proven to be the best way to prevent cancer cells from growing.. and the fact that I'm lean, strong and healthier than ever.. well, those are just very exciting perks!" ~ Amanda Riester

"A lot of people are very surprised that I can be as strong as I am on a mostly raw vegan diet. At this point, anyone that knows me knows I'm a vegan because I make a point to wear a VEGAN item every day. A tank, shorts, my purse... even my license plate reads VEGAN. I am very proud to be so strong and so healthy on a vegan diet. I pride myself on being an ambassador for the vegan lifestyle!" ~ Amanda Riester

Chapter 4- Why a Vegan Diet Increases Performance

With so many people who believe that meat protein is essential for the body in order to compete effectively in performance sports, what is the truth? Why are so many vegans among the top in the world in their respective sports? Will your performance increase by deciding to adopt to a vegan diet?

Ask the Gladiators!

So why did Gladiators choose the vegan route? While quite obviously we are unable to actually go and talk to an actual Roman Gladiator, science has started to do most of the work for us. Bones analyzed that came from a cemetery known to be the resting place of these arena fighters has shown that the average diet was free from meat but high in plants and grains. Evidence has also been found that they consumed a drink, which was created from the ashes of plants.

This drink was apparently a type of tonic used for boosting health and assisting in the recovery after training and fighting. The evidence shows that the ashes of plants appear to have been consumed due to their fortifying effects on the body. They helped to speed recovery after physical exertion and also to promote quicker healing of bones.

The Nutritional Advantage

From a nutritional viewpoint, vegan diets can easily provide all of the essential nutrients that are known to increase the effectiveness of strength training. Except of zinc and iron, scientific evidence is beginning to show that a vegan diet may even provide better nutrition than any other type of diet.

Protein is often what the majority of people assume to be missing in a vegan diet. While it is true that their protein does not come from animal sources, there are a number of available sources of protein for vegans. A varied and healthy vegan diet includes legumes, seeds, nuts, whole grain products, lots of leafy greens, vegetable, and fruits. The most common nutrients are listed below, minus protein, which will be discussed in more detail in the next chapter:

Calcium

Needed to build strong bones, calcium is found in orange juice, soymilk that has been fortified, tofu, dark green vegetables, almonds, and a variety of other common foods that vegans eat.

Vitamin D

Vitamin D is not found naturally in the vegan diet. 15 minutes of sun per day is sufficient to give the amount needed for the average adult, however. It can also be found in fortified rice milk and soy milk.

Fat

Since a vegan diet is low in saturated fat and free from cholesterol, the risk of many serious conditions and diseases can be greatly reduced by switching to a vegan diet. The body does need fat in moderation and vegans can find it in coconuts, avocados, seed butters, nut butters, nuts, and various oils.

Iron

Iron is essential for proper performance of athletes. On a per calorie basis, vegan sources of iron such as dark green leafy vegetables and dried beans are a better choice than meat. Absorption of iron is enhanced by consuming foods that contain Vitamin C at the same time. Good sources include prune juice, watermelon, kale, beet greens, chickpeas, blackstrap molasses, and lentils.

Omega-3 Fatty Acids

Most people think of Omega-3s as only being found in fish and seafood. However, vegans can easily find what they need in walnuts, soybeans, tofu, canola oil, flaxseed oil, and flax seeds.

The Benefits that are Noticeable Right Away

Aspiring athletes who make the switch to a vegan diet will notice many changes in their body and the way it reacts during training and competitions. One of the biggest benefits that athletes often feel almost instantly is how much more energy they have. This makes it easier to complete training schedules without becoming fatigued. One of the main reasons for this is quite simple.

Consider an athlete who eats a normal "Western" diet which contains dairy products and meat. These things are actually foreign to our bodies, and a huge amount of energy is expended trying to digest and utilize what has been consumed. This means that right off the bat these athletes have wasted a chunk of their valuable energy stores to process what was eaten. On the other hand, a vegan diet is easily absorbed, digested, and utilized by the body.

Another benefit that can be seen is how quickly the body will recover after intense exercise. Injuries are less likely to occur, and muscles and ligaments have all the nutrients they need to expand and move during complicated maneuvers.

There are so many benefits adopting a full vegan diet that it is impossible to do much more than touch them briefly throughout this book. One that must be mentioned, however, is how much easier it will be to not only to fall asleep at night, but also to stay asleep and wake up refreshed. While some meat eaters toss and turn during the body feverishly tries to digest unnatural food, many vegans slip right off to dreamland. Every athlete knows the importance of getting plenty of quality rest.

Popular Vegan Supplements

There are times when the body has increased needs, due to an intense training or competition schedule. It is for these times that supplements are an invaluable asset to athletes who want their performance to be at an all time high. Thankfully, there are many supplements that are appropriate for the vegan diet.

But how do supplements actually work? What happens when you swallow that pill? Simply put, the active ingredients contained within the supplement are released into the stomach after you swallow them. From here they pass through the small intestine before being distributed throughout the bloodstream. When the body breaks down the nutrients it is, when the majority of supplements fail. Stomach acids easily destroy poor-quality nutrient supplements, leaving you with an absorption rate of less than 10%. Choosing high-quality supplements is beyond essential!

The 4 Most Important Factors to Consider When Choosing Health Supplements

To make sure that you are getting the optimum results from your health supplements, pay attention to these 4 factors when you go shopping!

- **Bioavailability:** The higher the absorption rate of the supplement, the better it is. They are of no use to the body if no absorption occurs. Liquid nutritional supplements offer the best absorption rate.
- **All-Natural:** Look at the ingredient list carefully. Search for supplements which have no added artificial preservatives, allergens, or dyes. Keeping your supplements as all-natural as possible is the ultimate goal.

- **Tested in the Lab:** Reputable companies will stand behind their products and submit to testing done not only by their in-house labs, but also by independents.

Calcium

Calcium is essential for the formation of stronger bones that athletes in particular need. High-performance athletes put a huge amount of stress on their bones so, in order to ensure that breaks do not occur, calcium supplements are available in various strengths.

Iron

Iron can be a difficult mineral to get enough of. It is a part of every cell in the body and is responsible for carrying oxygen from the lungs to other parts of the body. This is a vital mineral for athletes.

Zinc

Athletes require zinc for numerous functions throughout the body, but mostly for proper workings of bones and muscles. The bioavailability of zinc, when obtained from plant sources is said to be less than from meat and dairy. To ensure that your body does not run out of this trace mineral, it is recommended for athletes that a supplement is taken.

Protein Powders

While plenty of protein can be found in the vegan diet, these powders are a good way to get some extra protein when it is needed quickly. For example in the morning or right after training. They mix easily with water or juice and are available in a number of flavors.

"B" Vitamins

There are 8 different groups of B-Vitamins, and they are more than essential for athletes since they are needed for energy production and red blood cell production. They are also known as the "stress" vitamin..

Vitamin C

While this may seem to be surprising, not all vegans are major fruit lovers. While fruit is known as the best source of Vitamin C, it is also prevalent in vegetables. Even though more than enough can be found in vegetables, in order to ensure that you are keeping up a steady supply in your body a supplement may be a good idea. There are several forms of Vitamin C available. Any extra Vitamin C that has been consumed, but not used by the body, will be excreted in the urine.

Chapter 5- Increasing Performance: Sports Nutrition Guidelines

Now that you fully understand exactly what a vegan diet can do for you, it is time for a chapter on the nutrition guidelines of what you need to eat in order to increase your performance in both training and competition. While all vitamins and minerals are essential for performance athletes, a great concern for the majority are the right amount/source of carbohydrates and protein.

Exercise is essential for health, and eating food that is healthy will help you get the most out of the exercise that you do. Nutritional deficiencies and poor eating habits can impair performance. Here are a few great meals and snacks that you should consider adding in so that you will shine:

Carbohydrates

Usually, carbohydrates are the primary fuel, which is utilized when you are doing high-intensity exercise. The carbohydrate needs for athletes are close to those for anyone else on a per-calorie basis (a minimum of 55% of your total daily intake of calories). More specific recommendations for athletes are done based primarily on weight, and they range on average from 6-10 grams per kilo of body weight each day. A staggering amount of evidence shows that the availability of carbohydrates boosts performance and endurance. Excellent sources of carbohydrates include vegetables, fruits, and whole grain foods. Depending on how much exercise is done and how strenuous the workout is, carbohydrate synthesis peaks 30 minutes to 2 hours post activity. Foods that are rich in carbohydrates and which have a moderate to high Glycemic index offer an easily available source for the production of glycogens.

Proteins

Chains of molecules known as amino acids are what proteins are composed of. They play a vital role in the repair, maintenance, and building of all the tissues in the body, including muscles. There are a total of 20 different amino acids, but only 11 of them can be produced by the body. Nine of these are essential amino acids and must be obtained from food. All of the essential amino acids can easily be provided by a diet containing a variety of vegetables, legumes, and whole grains. It had once been thought that various plant foods must be eaten at the same time to get all of their protein value. This method is known by either "complementing" or "protein combining"." Scientists found out, that it is not necessary to combine the full spectrum of amino acids in every meal, to have optimal muscle growth.

Athletes utilize protein primarily to rebuild and repair muscle that has broken down during physical activity. It is also used to help optimize glycogen storage. Protein isn't a great source of fuel during exercise, but it can be used when adequate carbohydrates are lacking in the diet. This is detrimental though,

because if protein is used as a fuel source, there could be a lack to rebuild and repair body tissues, especially muscle. So how much protein is needed?

- The average adult requires 0.8 grams daily per kilogram of body weight.
- Strength training athletes require roughly 1.4 to 1.8 grams daily per kilogram of body weight.
- Endurance athletes require roughly 1.2 to 1.4 grams daily per kilogram of body weight.

Athletes who are looking for quick sources of extra protein may want to consider some of the following:

- Instead of just eating a boring salad, try adding a mixture of various beans on top such as black beans, great northern beans, kidney beans, and chickpeas. These powerful legumes have as much as 7 -10 grams of protein in each serving.

- Make a shake! Blend together soft tofu or nondairy milks with your favorite frozen or fresh fruits for a deliciously thick and creamy high-protein "milk" shake.

- Marinated veggie or tempeh burgers can be grilled and added to pasta sauce or placed on a whole grain bun for a quick boost of protein.

- Snack on the run? Rice protein shakes and nutrition bars are a convenient and quick supplement to help increase the protein content of any vegan diet.

Water

Maintaining the optimal state of hydration is essential so that any athlete can operate at peak performance levels and reduce the incidences of injury. Dehydration, which is defined as a body weight loss of more than 1% due to loss of fluids, results in a variety of symptoms, including dark urine with a strong odor, heat intolerance, fatigue, and headache.

More serious side effects include heat stroke, heat exhaustion, heat cramps, and neuromuscular fatigue. By maintaining a regular schedule of fluid consumption that equals at least eight 8-ounce glasses of water every day, symptoms like these are prevented easily. Fluid needs increase with an increased amount of exercise. Also, keep in mind that participating in activities at high temperatures, in low humidity, or at high altitudes can also increase your body's need for fluid replacement.

Follow these general guidelines to make sure that the hydration is never a problem:

- Drink 2 cups (or about 14 to 20 ounces) of fluid two hours before exercise.
- Drink 1 to 1.5 cups (or about 5 to 12 ounces) of fluid every 15 to 20 minutes during exercise.
- Drink 2 to 3 cups (or about 16 to 24 ounces) of fluid after exercising for every pound that has been lost during physical exertion. Weigh yourself before and after in order to determine how much fluid you are losing.

Water is the perfect fluid replacer, especially during activities which last less than one hour. For other more intensive activities that last longer than 60 to 90 minutes, electrolyte or carbohydrate-containing sports drinks may be useful both during and after exercise.

Conclusion

Thank you again for downloading this book!

I hope this book helped you to learn about the ways in which a vegan diet will help you to become not only a better performing athlete, but also healthier overall.

The next step is to decide how and when you are going to make the switch. Whether you choose to do it slowly, or you prefer to just jump right in, the important thing is that you have made the decision. Within a short time, you should notice many positive changes and improvements in how your body feels and responds during periods of physical activity. You should see how much better you are able to train and compete as well as feel much better overall.

In the beginning, it may take a little bit of getting used to, once you have switched to the fully vegan diet. However, it will not take long for your body to eliminate all of the "bad stuff". Once this happens, you should notice that you have made the right decision, not only for your health, but also to improve your sports performance.

Finally, if you enjoyed this book, then I'd like to ask you for a favor and leave a review for this book on Amazon. It would be greatly appreciated!